Meet Bev. She's a superhero. You may have seen her before.
She likes to fly over the city, rescue cats from trees,
and pick trash out of the ocean.

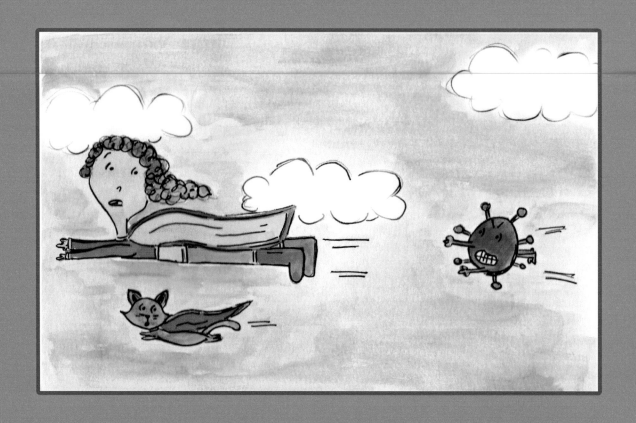

Now, even though Bev is a superhero, she can still get sick, just like the rest of us. While her superpowers may let her soar through the clouds, they do not protect her from germs!

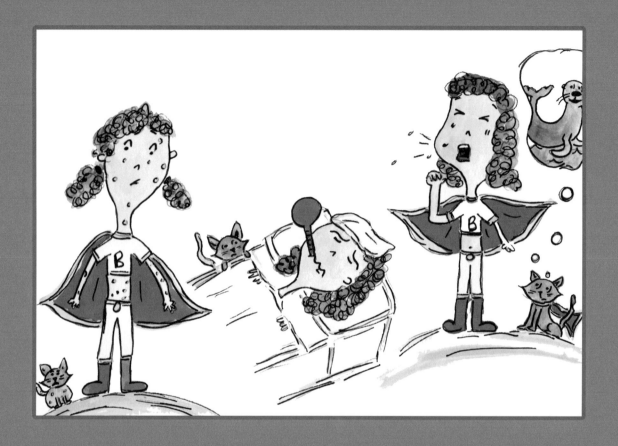

Bev could get a barking cough like a seal from a germ called Pertussis. She could get polka dot skin from the Measles. And she could run a fever as hot as the sun from Diptheria. And if Bev is sick, who will protect the ocean? Who will save the cats?

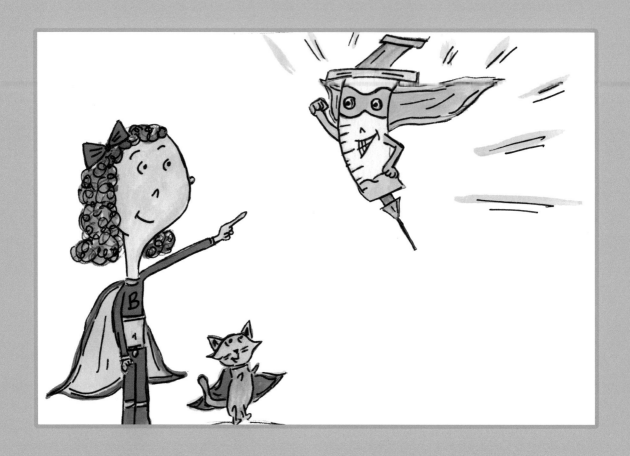

So, in order to keep herself healthy and safe, Bev gets her vaccines! Slow down you may say—what is a **vaccine**?

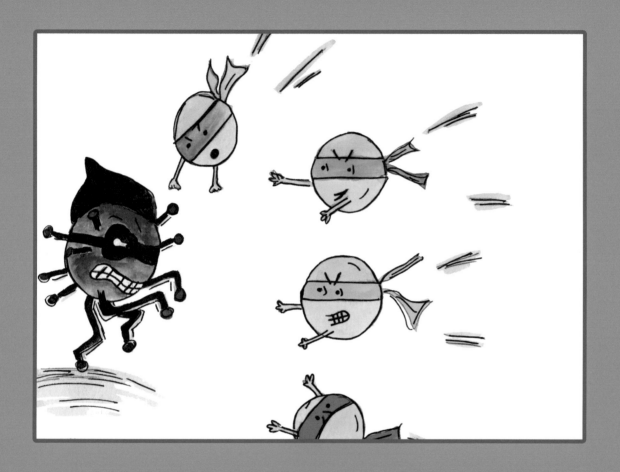

First, Bev must introduce you to the **immune system**.
Everyone, even Bev, has a group of superheroes that live
inside them. This is the immune system. The immune
system fights off bad guys called germs, like viruses or
bacteria, that sneak into our bodies.

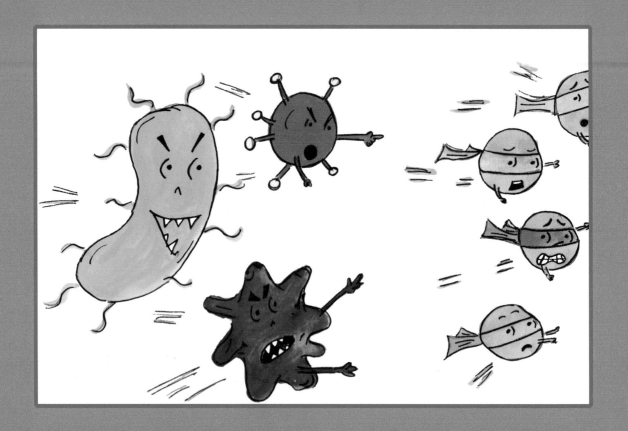

Sometimes these germs are so strong that our immune system needs help protecting us. Time to call in the vaccines!

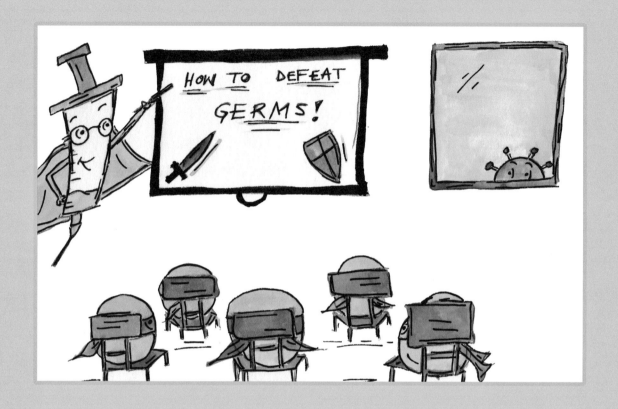

Vaccines are superhero masters who teach our immune system how to fight off the bad guys. This may sound crazy, but vaccines are actually made from parts of the bad germs. This gives them the secret information on how to defeat the bad germs. They then use this information to teach our immune system how to protect us. Just like a karate master teaching a beginner student how to deliver a strong POW!

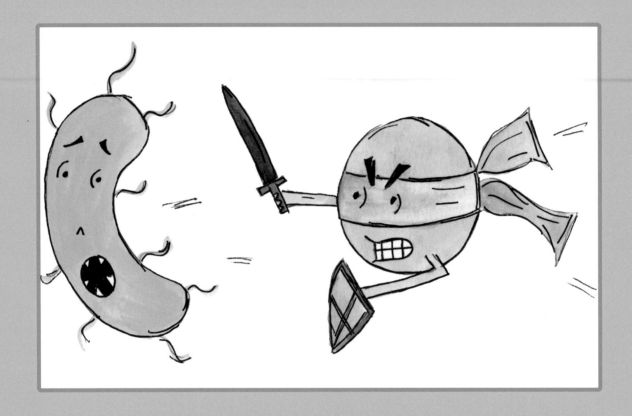

So, when the bad germs show up, our superhero immune system will be ready and can fight them off. Not only will you stay healthy and happy, but this will also keep you from spreading the bad germs to other people. It's like feeding two cats with one fish!

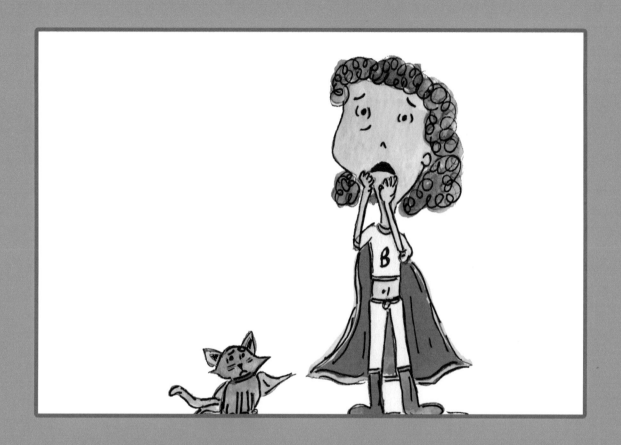

Even though Bev understands how important vaccines are, she can still feel a little nervous to get one. Will it hurt? Will it make her feel bad? Will it cause her arm to turn a funny color? Even superheroes get scared.

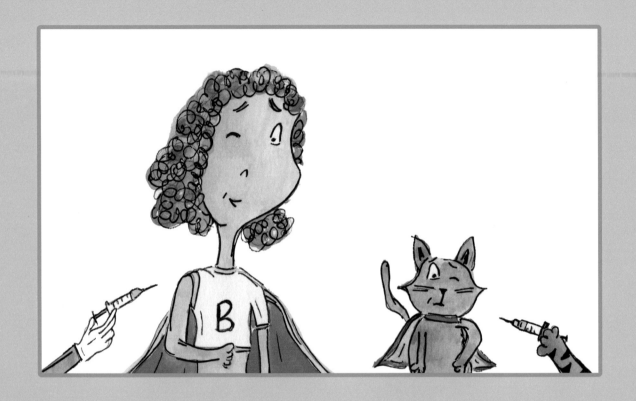

But then she remembers: It's just a tiny poke — like a baby bee sting. And while it may make her feel a little weak or blue for a day or two, it's just like feeling tired after training for a big karate match or soccer game. Definitely worth it.

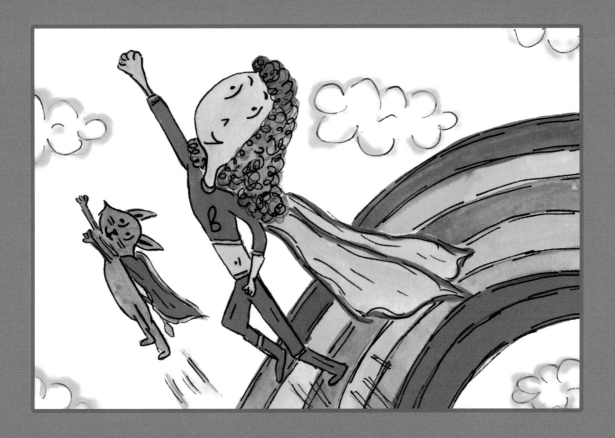

And most importantly, vaccines will protect her, her friends, her family, and people all over the world. Because vaccines help everyone become superhero protectors! Now let's fly!

MEET THE BAD GUYS

The Flu — We know it well. The Flu is a virus that attacks your nose, throat, and lungs causing a stuffy nose, headaches, and fevers. It spreads through mucus droplets (like when you sneeze, and it flies through the air! Ewwww...)

Diphtheria — This bacteria attacks our nose and throat, making our throats sore and sometimes even making it hard to breathe.

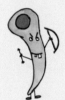

Tetanus — The tetanus bacteria lives in the soil and enters our body through cuts in our skin. It has a special weapon, which is a poison that makes our muscles tighten up and sometimes spasm or shake.

Pertussis — This bad guy causes whooping cough. Sounds silly but it gives you coughing fits like a barking seal. Not great when you are trying to watch a movie...

Rotavirus — This virus attacks our intestines, making us throw up and have lots of diarrhea.

Poliovirus — This bad guy is almost completely gone thanks to the Poliovirus vaccine. But it can attack people who have not been protected, causing paralysis in some cases (being unable to move your body). Interesting fact — Franklin Delano Roosevelt (the 32nd President of the United States) had polio, and became paralyzed from the waist down when he was 39 years old.

Measles — Also known as Rubeola, this bad guy can give you fevers and sore throat. It also causes tiny little white spots to appear in your mouth, and causes your skin to get a bright red blotchy rash. Thankfully, it is very rare because of its vaccine!

Mumps — The Mumps likes to attack lots of parts of your body, but its favorite places are the saliva glands in your mouth called the parotid (not parrot) glands. It brings on fevers, headaches, and puffy cheeks from swollen parotid glands.

Rubella — This virus causes a red rash and mild symptoms, but can be more dangerous to pregnant women, and can spread to and harm brand new babies. Thankfully, this is rare because of its vaccine!

Haemophilus influenza type b (Hib) — This is a really bad bacteria that can hurt our brain, throat, and lungs.

Varicella — The chickenpox! Also known as the 'very itchy bad guy.' Causes an itchy rash of blisters.

Hepatitis A & B — These viruses like to attack our livers, and we need our livers! Sometimes they even turn our skin and eyes yellow and cause belly pain.

Streptococcus pneumoniae — This bacteria can hurt our brain, lungs, and ears. It can cause a cold, an ear infection, or make our brain swollen and angry.

Meningococcus — This super bad guy attacks our brains and can travel through our blood. It is very mean and dangerous.

Human papillomavirus — This virus can cause cancers later in life so it's important to learn to protect ourselves early from it!

COVID-19 — I'm sure you have heard about this virus. This bad guy went crazy and hurt a lot of people by attacking lungs, and sometimes other organs too. It has not hurt kids as badly as adults, but can be more dangerous if you have underlying health issues like diabetes or asthma.

MEET THE SUPERHERO MASTERS

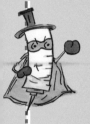

Flu vaccine — a special shot or nasal spray that protects us from the flu. The flu virus mutates (or changes) every year. So, the vaccine changes every year to teach us the newest protections! Kids can get the flu vaccine starting at age 6 months. Make sure to get it every year! The vaccine can cause some of us to feel not so hot after. But remember, it is because your immune system is preparing for battle!

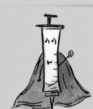

DTaP vaccine — a series of 5 vaccine shots that protect us from 3 bad guys (diphtheria, tetanus, and pertussis). These shots protect us for 10 years. Given at age 2, 4, 6, 15–18 months, and 4–6 years.

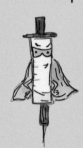

Tdap vaccine — a shot that 'boosts' the power of the DTaP vaccine given at age 11 years old (like a superhero sidekick).

Rotavirus vaccine — a shot given in several doses to protect us from Rotavirus starting at age 2, 4, and 6 months.

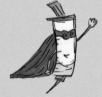

IPV vaccine — a special superhero vaccine that protects us from polio. Comes as four different training lessons (or shots) at age 2, 4, 6–18 months, and 4–6 years.

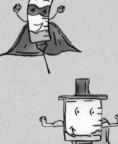

MMR vaccine — a really strong superhero master that protects us from 3 bad guys (measles, mumps, and rubella). We get 2 training sessions with this vaccine at age 12–15 months and then again at age 4–6 years.

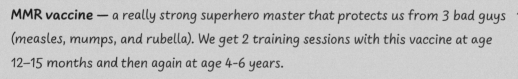

Hib vaccine — a series of 3 or 4 shots given at age 2, 4, 6, and 12– 15 months to prevent Haemophilus influenzae type B.

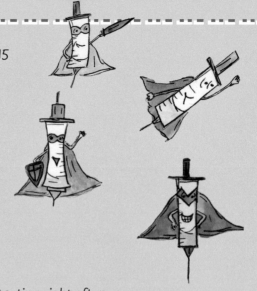

Hepatitis A vaccine — a series of 2 shots given between age 12-23 months, 6 months apart.

Varicella vaccine — a vaccine to protect us from the itchiest of bad guys (chickenpox). We get this at age 12-15 months and then again at age 4-6 years.

HBV vaccine — this superhero vaccine gives us 3 training lessons starting right after we're born to help protect our liver from hepatitis B. We get 3 doses total at age 0, 1–2, and 6–18 months.

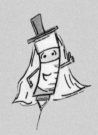

Pneumococcal vaccine — a series of 4 vaccine shots at age 2, 4, 6, and 12–15 months.

Meningococcal vaccine — a very important superhero vaccine that protects our brains. This training takes place as 2 shots at age 11-12 years and at age 16 years.

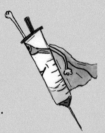

HPV vaccine — a superhero master shot that protects us from the human papillomavirus, which can cause cancers later in life. It is a series of 2 or 3 shots starting at age 9-12 years old.

COVID-19 vaccine — I'm sure you've heard about this superhero master! This vaccine protects us from COVID-19 and can help to protect our families and friends. We can get one or more doses starting at age 6 months. Check with your doctor to see if you are up to date or need an updated 'booster' shot.

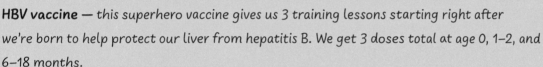

Vaccine Schedule

	Birth	1 month	2 months	4 months	6 mont
The Flu					✦
DTaP			✦	✦	✦
Meningococcus					
Rotavirus			✦	✦	✦
Polio (IPV)			✦	✦	
MMR					
HiB			✦	✦	✦
Varicella					
Hepatitis B	✦	✦			
Pneumococcus			✦	✦	✦
HPV					

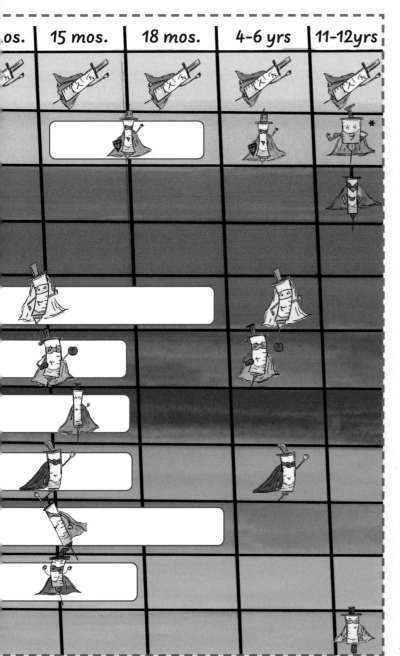

os.	15 mos.	18 mos.	4-6 yrs	11-12yrs

*Tdap vaccine

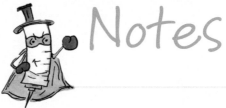

Notes

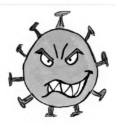

Hepatitis A vaccine
is given between ages
12 and 23 months as 2 doses,
6 months apart.

Get your **COVID-19** vaccine
starting at age 6 months and up!

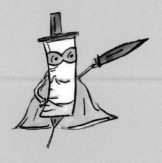

Facts

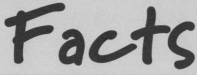

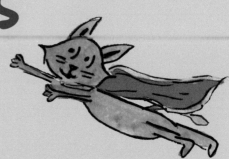

1. Vaccines are safe.

2. It is MUCH safer to get a vaccine than to get the disease.

3. Vaccines have made many serious childhood diseases rare today—like polio, mumps, and measles.

4. Without vaccines, these diseases could return and hurt a lot of people.

5. Some people with severe allergies to vaccines or certain cancers or immune system diseases cannot get vaccines. This makes it even more important for the people who can get vaccines to get them because of **herd immunity**.

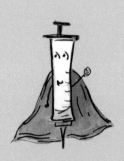
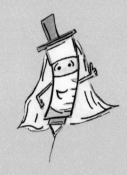
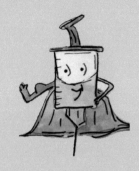

6. **Herd immunity** is when a lot of people are vaccinated against a disease and it protects a whole group of people (even ones who are not vaccinated) because it makes the spread of the disease very rare.

7. Side effects from vaccines are usually very mild and can include a fever, general body aches, and soreness at the shot site.

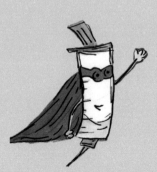

8. Research shows that there is NO link between autism and childhood vaccines.

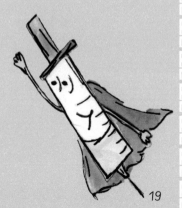

Meet the Author:

Dr. Maria Baimas-George

Maria Baimas-George MD MPH is a surgeon, training to specialize in abdominal transplantation. Inspired by her patients and mentors, she writes and illustrates books explaining medical and surgical conditions to children and their loved ones. Her goal is to create books that provide useful information to help with understanding and to offer comfort and hope.

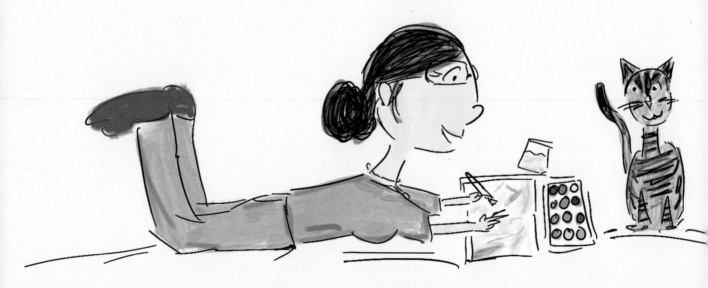